The Hangover Handbook: 15 Natural Cures To Knock Out Your Hangover Quickly & Effectively

Disclaimer and Terms of Use: Effort has been made to ensure that the information in this book is accurate and complete, however, the author and the publisher do not warrant the accuracy of the information, text and graphics contained within the book due to the rapidly changing nature of science, research, known and unknown facts and internet. The Author and the publisher do not hold any responsibility for errors, omissions or contrary interpretation of the subject matter herein. This book is presented solely for motivational and informational purposes only.

Table of Contents

Introduction

Hangover refers to the experience of some of the unpleasant psychological and physiological effects which are resultant of alcohol consumption. It is featured with a discomfort feeling that is very severe which can last up-to one day. Normally, some of the common symptoms that are resultant of hangover include concentration problems, headaches, dry mouth, drowsiness, anxiety, hyper-excitability, nausea, sweating, gastrointestinal complaints, fatigue and dizziness.

This guide has been designed to give you the 15 best ways of overcoming hangovers effectively and in the most efficient ways. With this you will have both the pre-drinking and post-drinking ideas that will help you cure a hangover after your alcoholic beverage intake. They are more than remedies in that you will have ways which are natural to control your hangover and get rid of it. Normally you will hear people saying that, "They will never drink ever again" after waking up after a night they spent drinking. In this case most people experience some of the mentioned symptoms which are severe including headaches as well as stomach rolling.

Drinking Water Before And While Drinking.

This is the first remedy and very simple, although very important to reduce your hangover that you might have encountered the next day. Prior to heading to the partying ceremony, bash, rave or even other activities that entails a lot of drinking you should ensure that you have drank plenty of water which will assist in keeping your body hydrated as well as assist in dilution of the alcohol that you will have taken. Actually it is also advisable to dilute your alcoholic beverage with water or soft drinks as they contain a lot of water. This reduces the alcohol concentration in your blood and body.

This should also be done the next morning after your drinking activity. You can also consider taking electrolyte-replenishing sports drinks. They highly assist in easing any symptoms that might result from dehydration that normally go hand-in-hand with hangovers. According to health research in the process of breaking down alcohol in the body for absorption purposes there is production of chemicals like lactic acid that have great interferences in the sugar and glucose production as well as electrolytes in the body. This is the reason why intake of sports drinks can be highly recommended. You should never drink any drinks that have caffeine in them like coffee due to the fact that they have great contribution in dehydration.

Water will also assist you to visit the toilet or urinal many times which are a great tools of reducing the concentration of alcohol in the body. Generally it is very easy to know that a drunken person had used the urinal before you when you visit it. This is due to the fact that some of the alcohol impurities that were not absorbed by the blood and body are discharged out of the body as waste. Water will assist lowering the concentration of the same by making you urinate as many times as possible. Actually it is highly recommended to drink around eight glasses of water in the morning in case you are feeling severe hangover symptoms.

Again consumption of alcohol results into dehydration due to the fact that alcohol causes you to have a loss of more water from the body than you had taken through the stimulation of the kidneys.

Consider Eating Something That Contains A Lot Of Fat.

Prior to the partying event or before the drinking spree, consider eating foods which have a lot of fat contents. The logic behind this is the fact that as opposed to most of the carbohydrates, fats slows the absorption rates of alcohol in your body and blood. You can choose to use fried foods, sausage, steak as well as pizza prior to your partying activity. According to the heath research, fats sit in your body and the intestines linings for more than 12 hours which gives room for slow rates of alcohol absorption into the blood and body. This will reduce the alcohol that would have entered your blood thus reducing hangovers.

Consider Spacing The Intervals Of Your Drinks.

This means that you should not drink throughout, that is bottle after bottle or glass after glass of drinks, rather it is important to have some break between the respective drinks. In this time of break you can opt to take soft drinks, water or even chat with friends. This will offer dilution of the alcohol that you will have taken in your body. In case you are a teenager or young in a party you can dance or even walk around to relax your body prior to the next drink.

Stick To Alcoholic Drinks Which Are Light.

Consider the usage and intake of the alcoholic drinks which are light. These are in inclusion of the clear liquors like gin and vodka as well as beer. In any case if you want to reduce and remedy hangovers effectively consider not drinking dark/malt liquors like rum and whiskey as well as the red wine which has higher effects of hangovers. This is due to the fact that the latter drinks have got tannins which results to high hangover effects.

Consider Taking A Non-Acetaminophen Over-The Counter Pain Killer Like Aspirin.

This should be in the morning after the drinking event. You should not take a pain killer in the night you were drinking due to the fact that their effects in the body last for only four hours and thus they won't help you in the morning. Thus, you should take it in the morning after your drinking spree. Actually alcohol and alcoholic beverages have a disruption on how your liver processes the acetaminophen. Thus, you should not take any pain killer that has got acetaminophen as it can lead to permanent damage or inflammation of the liver.

Taking some medications like zofran and vioden can also highly assist in this case. With it you will have a chance of upsetting your stomach as well as feeling reborn. Although you are highly advised never to use Tylenol as it will worsen the situation. Taking pain relievers is a very good idea in case you are waking up for work the morning after a long night of drinking. Alcohol results in the widening of your blood vessels, this causes a lot of pain in the brain that results into a lot of headaches. Whereas they will not assist you to get better or offer you with any kind of treatment, pain relievers highly assist in making you have a better feeling for a short duration and thus be able to concentrate with your work.

Eating Toasts That Have Been Burnt.

To assist in filtration of impurities that result from alcohol drinking, the carbons from the parts of the toast which have been burnt are very helpful. This is the reason why many people who end up being hospitalized due to alcohol poisoning are pumped with carbon slurry inside their stomachs.

You should also consider eating foods which are bland like crackers and toast. These foods do not assist in absorbing the alcohol but rather they help in boosting your blood sugar. Generally, alcohol and alcoholic beverages results in prevention of blood sugar concentration in your body, this can result into weaknesses and fatigue due to the low levels of blood sugar inside your body. You may also consider taking complex carbohydrates like bread and cereals which are great choices.

You can also consider making a bacon sandwich. The bread which is inherent in the sandwich will assist in raising the levels of your blood sugar whereas the proteins which are inside the bacon highly assist in breaking down the amino acids that helps in the replenishment of neurotransmitters of the brain that might have depleted through the alcohol intake. Eating of plain-starchy foods also gives you another advantage. These are in inclusion of crackers, toast, as well as plain bagels which are very great when taken during the instances of hangovers. They are not sweet and tasty when eating but very well in replenishing your blood sugars.

Consider Having Bouillon Soup For Storing Potassium And Salt.

Potassium is a very important mineral when it comes to muscles and nerve functions, although it is highly lost in the urination process after alcohol drinking. Thus it is very vital to consider taking in foods which have potassium and salts to regain the lost levels of their concentration in the body. Consider taking in avocados, glass of orange juice, potato chips as well as bananas to help in potassium restoration in the body.

You should also consider the intake of foods and drinks that have fructose. Such foods highly assist in burning the alcohol faster. This is a great remedy that you should impose the next morning after your drinking spree. Actually this can be achieved by eating fruits as well as fruit juices which have high fructose content to assist you in feeling better. Generally, fructose does not assist in easing the symptoms which are related to the hangover but rather they highly assist in easing the alcohol metabolic effects.

Be Happy And Chewing Ginger.

"Being happy" is a phrase which sounds very simple although it is a very important act in hangover reduction. Actually characteristics like being highly depressed or angry after drinking, having neurotic personalities, having guilt after alcohol intake or even have negative feelings after the drinking spree results in high chances of the hangover symptoms. They are even more severe than what or how much you had drank. Thus, it is very important to ensure that you are happy and in good moods after drinking to ensure that you have countered any negative feeling that might have resulted from not being in a good mood.

Chewing ginger will also assist you in reducing the hangover. You can consider chewing small pieces of ginger but alternatively you can boil around 10 pieces of ginger roots which are fresh in about three-to-four cups of water, you should then add some orange juice, lemon juice as well as a tablespoon of honey. This mixture actually highly assists in quick relief from the hangover through stabilization of the levels of your blood glucose.

Eating Eggs As Well As Having Ample Sleep.

Eggs have got high contents of amino acids which are called Cysteine; they help in countering acetaldehyde effects that result from alcohol intake and are known to have high rates of hangover creations. Thus, eggs intake will highly assist in reduction of hangovers at the long-run.

On the other hand sleeping acts as one of the most essential and effective ways of treating hangovers this is due to the fact that your body will not get a chance of going through the "rapid-eye-movement". In the sleeping state your brain will have an ample time to restore glutamine and will rebound inside your body.

In case your hangovers are severe consider going back to sleep. You may have drank a lot, such that even the time that you slept was not ample to assist you in not getting to the R.E.M. during which your body restores itself. In such an instance you should consider crawling back to your bed and have some more sleep. Ensure that you have wrapped yourself in the blanket. You can also put on some music which will soothe you to sleep. In case you are a student or work you can call the admin and state that you are "Sick" although "DON'T-DO-THIS" routinely.

Consumption Of Soothing Foods.

Consumption of soothing foods highly relives your body from rolling. These foods have to contain high vitamin content that will replenish the store of your vitamins in the body. As mentioned above you can consider the intake of foods like bananas and apples which have got high nutrient contents. They will offer elimination of headaches and other related symptoms through the restoration of minerals, more so the potassium mineral.

Consumption of tomatoes also assists in revitalizing and refreshing you. You should consider slicing them and have some addition of pepper and salt. This fruit has a high fructose content that helps in the metabolism of alcohol in the body. To heighten the results you can add some lime juice in it. Coconut eating further assists in potassium restoration in the body. Actually after drinking alcohol potassium is the salt that you highly lose during the urination and sweating process; whereas it is very important in muscles and nerves working. You can also drink coconut water. You can consider cabbage intake as well. This should either be done by eating fresh-raw cabbages or extracting its juice and adding it to the tomato juice. It really helps in stabilization of the blood glucose.

Consumption Of Soothing Drinks.

As mentioned, consider drinking revitalizing drinks. This highly helps in rehydration of your body which is a key area in the fight against hangovers. Some of them also help in restoration of electrolytes and settling of your stomach quicker than others. Drinking flat-ginger ale can also do more. Actually this helps in soothing your stomach. It is important to understand that stomach disorders can be felt in the head through headaches. Drinking pedialyte which has got very low sugar contents and high sodium content also assists in rehydration of your body. Actually this drink tastes very good along with being rich in vitamins. This can serve you better than the soft and sports drinks.

Munching on some ice-pops and taking them can be a great idea in case you are not feeling like drinking. It assists in the rehydration process as well as assisting you from the bloated felling. Drinking juice can also be a very great idea. Juices have got high vitamin contents that will assist in replenishing cravings that you have. You can consider taking pineapple, mango, orange as well as any other fruit juice. While taking the drinks ensure that you are doing it slowly.

Usage Of Herbal Remedies.

Trying some herbal remedies is a great natural way of remedying hangovers. These remedies highly help in replenishment of the lost nutrients. The first herbal remedy can be the use of milk thistle. This can be a great recommendation to the people who have hangovers and are associated with liver problems. If you are one of the affected individuals consider purchasing the tea or pills of milk thistle.

Another herbal method of remedying hangover is by the use of honey. This is the gift of bees to mankind. It highly helps in the treatment of hangovers through replenishment of the fructose levels. You can do it by adding some honey to boiling water thus making it more diluted as well as less sweet prior to consuming it.

Lemon can also do better. This helps in the detoxification of your body. You can do it through the preparation of some lemon tea and consume it which will in turn offer detoxification of your body. The other way is through chewing some ginger which will offer settling of your stomach. As discussed ginger candies are available in the store which can be consumed in small pieces.

You can also consider boiling around four to six leaves of crushed thyme in water. You should simmer this mixture for about 5 minutes and after the process strain the tea and drink while warm. This is actually a healthy and natural way of relieving hangovers. The thyme leaves assist in soothing your aching-muscles which is a great side effect of hangovers. It also helps in settling your stomach.

Another herbal way to relieve a hangover is through the use of activated charcoal-pills. Understand that you should not just crush the charcoal remnants that you have around the house, but rather you should find some charcoal pills at the local pharmacy. Charcoal which has been activated acts as an absorbent that assists in attracting the molecules which reband and then carries them away from the body.

Using Vitamins To Remedy Hangover.

Taking vitamin B-pills can be a very great way to remedy the hangover. By particularly taking vitamin B12 which is known as Cobalamin, you will have played a very large part in the functioning of the nervous system as well as the brain. You can boost your body in this way through the intake of supplements which have got high vitamin B contents. You can also achieve this through the intake of foods which are rich in vitamin B. Some of them includes citrus foods like oranges, cold milk as well as wheat.

Taking Vitamin-C pills which acts as an antioxidant can be a very great idea, this is due to the fact that the intake of alcohol results in the depression of your immunity. It is through this way that you expose your body to other viruses and colds that might result to hangovers. The use of vitamin C-antioxidants highly helps in fighting radicals which are free in our body thus alleviating headaches. Consider using Emergen-C as well as other flavored and powered vitamin C, which are very great in raising your vitamin C levels in the body. You can also consider taking drinks which taste like it.

Supplement taking will also serve you better. These are in inclusion of n-acetylcysteine that acts through the replenishing of your stores that have been depleted. You can also consider taking N-acetylcysteine that acts against the acetaldehyde that is a very great root-cause of hangovers.

Dealing With The Hangover.

You can remedy hangover by dealing with it. This is achievable in many ways. One of these ways includes sleeping and laying still. As noted before sleeping, drinking water, and having some time are the known ways to cure and remedy hangovers. In case you are finding it very hard to sleep you can consider putting your favorite movie or music that will relax you and then start closing your eyes. Although you might feel like the world is spinning, this is the best way to recover from a hangover.

The other way is getting along with some exercises which are light. In case you find it very hard to sleep take this step and have some bits of exercises. You can consider going on a brisk walk, swim or even jog to keep your brain awake and properly functioning. Exercises assist in boosting of your endorphins, this in turn helps in getting you from the black mood that is associated with the hangover. In any case through exercises your body becomes active thus metabolizing the alcohol in your body which relives the hangovers.

The other way to remedy a hangover naturally is through avoidance of loud noise as well as bright light. It is through hangovers that your increase in sensitiveness to sound and light is amplified. For you to have minimization of the pain involved you should start by closing your blinds and avoiding music which is loud, from there you should place a wash-cloth which is cool on your head. In case you want to get out you can wear a hat or sun glasses.

Taking a bath or shower is the other guaranteed way to counter a hangover. Although this method does not assist in remedying hangovers, it is highly recommended to make you feel better. Actually to soothe the stomach you can consider bathing with hot water.

Minimization Of Future Hangovers.

This is the last step although most important in this guide. After you have successfully alleviated the hangover it is good to put up means of minimizing hangovers in the future. One of the best and immediate ways is through the control of what and how you drink. While drinking it is good to stop and go when you feel you are buzzed. This is the best and immediate way to control your future as you will have trained your body on how much you can drink rather than drinking continuously.

Eating prior, after as well as during the drinking process is also a great idea. This assists you in keeping your sugar levels up which is also a very important way of hangover prevention. Drinking while your stomach is empty is a good ticket to a hangover as well as a cheap drink that might result to conditions which are more severe than the hangover. Consider the intake of foods which will assist you in the absorption of the alcohol that you will have drank. Actually having the intake of snacks throughout the night will reduce the hangovers that you would have felt the next day.

Drinking a lot of water throughout the night, after, or during a drinking spree can highly assist you. This will ensure that you have stayed hydrated which is a great way of hangover prevention. Alternatively, as mentioned early you can consider taking in a glass of water between the respective alcoholic drinks. In any case consider taking in two or three glasses of water prior to going to bed. You can also substitute the water with green tea which is also a great tool for hydrating your body and a better way of hangover prevention.

Avoidance of sugary and mixed drinks, this will lead to more hangovers instead of reducing it. You should ensure that you have avoided drinks which are made with mixes that are store bought, there are in inclusion of corn syrup as well as the sweet and sour mixes. Again understand the fact that sparkling wine has got high sugar contents. You can also consider taking in vitamin B prior to going to bed.

www.ingramcontent.com/pod-product-compliance
Lightning Source LLC
Chambersburg PA
CBHW072016280526
45788CB00005B/2073